In Search

of Truth

In Search

of Truth

Ridgeway Publishing
Medina, New York

IN SEARCH OF TRUTH

To order additional copies
please visit your local
bookstore or contact:

Ridgeway Publishing
3129 Fruit Avenue
Medina, NY 14103
ph: (888) 822-7894
fax: (585) 798-9016

ISBN# 978-0-9831460-1-8

Printed In the United States of America

Introduction

This is the poignant, personal story of one Amish couple's search of truth regarding the alternative medicine practice of *braucha*. While names and certain details have been changed to protect identity, the experiences are actual happenings.

As the publisher, it is our desire to help others become more aware of dangers that accompany some of these practices. May God receive all glory for any good that comes from this book.

Table of Contents

Chapter One

In Search of Truth

"Wa! Waaaaa!" The baby's insistent cry drew John King's attention away from his bookwork as he pushed his chair back from the desk.

"Here, give her to me," said John to his tired wife Mary, who had been trying to quiet one of the twins for at least the last half hour.

"I just don't know what could be wrong with these twins. They're so fussy every evening about this time," Mary said, subconsciously looking at the clock. "It's about time for their feeding. I guess we should take them to the doctor and find out if they have colic."

"I can tell Ruth has a stomachache," replied John as he laid his hands across the baby's belly.

"How can you tell?" asked Mary, not looking up as she filled the twins' bottles with goat milk. It seemed nothing else agreed with them.

"Just holding my hands on her stomach makes my stomach hurt a little," replied John.

"Do you think you could *brauch?*" questioned Mary, not really giving it any serious thought.

"Well, I don't know if I could or not, but it would be rather nice sometimes to be able to relieve them of their misery," answered John.

"It would save us some doctor bills too." Mary thought of their other four children. Every time they went to the doctor, it cost them $50 to $75, and sometimes more. With John just starting a repair shop, most of their money was tied up there.

"My grandfather used to be able to *brauch,*" John said thoughtfully, trying to remember incidents from a number of years before. "We were never allowed to watch, and I often wondered what he did. He always went into his bedroom, and sometimes he took a string and an egg along. After he was done he would throw the egg into the stove, and it would really pop. Usually the child would become well soon thereafter."

"Do you think he got this power from God?" asked Mary.

"Where else would you think it would come from? Surely you don't think an evil power could heal someone, do you?" questioned John.

"Well, I don't suppose so, but why would he have to use string and an egg to heal someone? I wonder if Scripture could shed any light on the subject?" Mary said, handing John a bottle.

"Lately I have had a hard time concentrating when reading the Bible, and yet I have no problem staying awake when I read the daily paper. Do you think we are spiritually drifting from the truth?" John asked. "I notice it is harder to keep my mind from wandering when we pray. Why, last night when I read the prayer, I even lost my place. I was so ashamed of myself. I wondered if God even hears such prayers!"

"What does that have to do with *braucha?*" Mary asked.

"I don't know if there's any connection or not, but I think it's worth looking into," John answered.

"Why don't we take the twins down to Jake Stoltzfus. He *brauchs* for a lot of children. Then we could ask him some questions. Surely he would know whether it's good or evil," concluded Mary.

Chapter Two

More Questions

The next evening after the shop was closed and the chores done, they hitched up old Rex to the buggy and drove several miles down the road to the Jake Stoltzfus home. As they turned in the lane, they noticed there were no other buggies. "Good," mused John. "Maybe if no one else is here we can ask Old Jake some questions."

John tied the horse, walked to the door, and knocked.

"Come on in," Jake said in his jolly way. "Cold out there, isn't it?"

"Yes, the evenings are getting quite chilly, although it's nice not to have so many mosquitoes," added John.

"What can we do for you tonight?" inquired Jake, chuckling a little.

"Ah, we thought maybe you would have time to *brauch* for our twins," replied John.

"Sure! What seems to be the problem?" Jake asked, cocking his head a little to get the babies' attention.

"Well, they seem quite colicky." Mary spoke up for the first time. "Ruth seems worse than Ruby, so maybe you could take her first." For some reason she felt uncomfortable in Jake's presence.

"Bring her over here on the couch," motioned Old Jake, who wasn't as old as he looked. He walked as if his feet hurt him and with a hunched back that made him look older than his late fifties.

Mary carried Ruth across the room and laid her on the couch, standing nearby in case Ruth started to cry. Old Jake came out of the bedroom rubbing his hands. Kneeling in front of the couch, he laid both hands on Ruth's stomach. Mary and John watched closely and noticed his lips moving.

Thinking he was praying, they silently bowed their heads, only to be disturbed by Jake's movements. Now Old Jake was moving his hands, starting at Ruth's head and moving on down her body, across her legs, and off her feet, shaking his hands vigorously as he reached the end. He did this three times. His hands shook and perspiration ran down his cheeks, even though John and Mary were just comfortable with their outer wraps still on.

"Well," said Old Jake, groaning as he straightened, "this one has quite a bellyache. I think we'll try something else on her yet." Walking over to the sewing machine, he took a spool of thread from the drawer. He measured out a piece of string Ruth's length. Tying the ends in a knot, he made a complete circle. Then he stood little Ruth on her feet and asked Mary to hold her. Not knowing what else to do, Mary followed his directions. He slipped the string over Ruth's body, again starting at the top and ending at the feet, three times.

Finally John couldn't contain himself any longer. "What is the purpose of this string?" he asked.

"Well, I really don't know how it works," admitted Old Jake, "but I'll take this string and wrap it around an egg and burn it. If the child is quite sick, the egg will burst with a loud noise, not even burning the string until the egg is popped."

"Where, ah . . ." stammered John, not knowing just how to word his question. "Where does this power come from? I mean, how does one get such a gift of healing?"

"Well," drawled Old Jake, stroking his beard, "I don't know where this power really comes from, but I certainly hope it is good." He seemed a little reluctant, but went on to say, "The gift is passed on when someone wants to quit. A man has to pass it on to a younger woman, or a woman to a younger man."

"What really is *braucha?*" inquired John, more curious all the time.

"Some people call it powwow," answered Jake, taking Ruby from John and laying her on the couch. "An older lady who wanted to quit gave me all the sayings and showed me how to do the different types of treatments. No one else is supposed to know the sayings. In fact, my wife doesn't even know them. Only when I am ready to quit may I expose these sayings, but then I have to quit practicing for good."

"Are stomachaches and such the only things that can be healed?" asked Mary.

"Oh, no!" Jake exclaimed. "The remedy for warts, for example, is to wait until full moon. Then, looking up at the moon, you rub your warts and say, 'What I see will add on; what I rub will take off.' Do this three times, and in a few days your warts will disappear. I have actually seen this happen. It really works, but you have to believe in it!"

Jake turned back to Ruby and performed the same ritual on her that he had on Ruth. "Here you go," said Jake, handing a crying Ruby back to John. "I can't do to much with them when they cry so hard, although I'm sure it will help some. Take this string home and hang it on the south wall, then put Ruth through it three times again for three days."

"South wall!" exclaimed John. "Why the south wall? After all, the sun goes down in the west, doesn't it?"

"Yes, it does at that," laughed Jake. "But the south wall is what they always said."

"We should be going," suggested John, nodding

to Mary for her approval. "I hope I didn't offend you with all my questions. What do we owe you for your time?"

Jake replied, "Oh, not much, just whatever you feel like."

John reached into his pocket for his wallet, searched for a few bills, and handed them to Jake.

"Thank you," said Jake. "Hope everyone will be better now. Good night."

"Good night," answered both John and Mary.

Chapter Three

Finding Some Answers

Neither spoke for a while, as they were both in deep thought. Finally Mary broke the silence. "John, what are you going to do with that string?"

"Well, one thing's for sure," mused John, "I won't hang that thing on the south wall. As soon as we get home, it will go into the stove. This is too much like . . . like, I don't know what! Something just isn't right!"

A few days later a customer came into the shop. It was a Mennonite man whom John vaguely knew.

"Good morning, Mr. Martin—Albert, I believe, isn't it?" greeted John.

"Yes, and how are you all?" Albert drawled.

"Just fine, and you?" replied John.

"Quite well, except a couple of the children have been fighting a round of flu or something. We had them down to Old Jake to see if he could help them," remarked Albert.

"Did it do any good?" questioned John. "I didn't know you believe in *braucha.*"

"I don't know that I really believe in it, although the Bible teaches about laying on of hands, doesn't it?" Albert asked.

"Yes, it does. In fact I'm just in the process of studying more on this subject," answered John. "We went to Old Jake a couple evenings ago with our twin girls, and I questioned him about *braucha.* It looks like a questionable procedure, and I haven't found any biblical evidence that this is the scriptural way of healing."

"I have wondered about it too. Maybe I'll check into it," replied Albert as he left the shop, leaving John in deep thought.

A few weeks later Albert returned to pick up his

repaired parts. After paying his bill, he again opened the subject of *bracha*. "Since our last visit," Albert started, "I bought a book that sheds some light on the subject. It's called *Between Christ and Satan*, by Kurt Koch, who is a Christian counselor in Germany. He has counseled thousands of people who have been involved with witchcraft and the occult."

"Would you actually say this is a form of witchcraft?" questioned John. "Surely Satan would not be able to heal, would he?"

"Kurt calls it white magic or mesmerism—the good side of Satan," Albert answered. "The real bad is called black magic."

"Do you mean Satan has a good side too?" asked John. "I always thought of him as all evil."

"Well, he is all evil as far as that goes, but the Bible also speaks of Satan being transformed into an angel of light and his ministers into ministers of righteousness."

"How can we tell if it is white magic or not? Old Jake said some people call it powwow." Thinking for a moment whether he should go on or not, John finally said, "I looked up in the dictionary what powwow means, and it described a ceremony of North American Indians, usually accompanied by magic, feasting, and dancing, performed for the cure of disease, success in hunting, victory in wars, or other purposes. Also, the word could be used to as a verb. A shaman or medicine man would powwow, meaning 'use divination.' "

"Okay, let's go back to Satan's good side," suggested Albert. "I believe Satan is the cause of all sickness. Let me explain. If Adam and Eve (or anyone else) had never sinned, then no one would ever have become sick, right?" Seeing John's nod of agreement, Albert went on. "If he can cause sickness, why would it be any harder to take it away? Look at Job. God allows sickness for various reasons and gives us the answer to healing in James 5, if we only obey and believe.

"Really, Satan doesn't have a good side to him, it only appears that way," Albert continued. "But in the end, it never turns out good. The works of Satan hinder our Bible reading and prayer. But Bible reading and prayer hinder the works of Satan."

With that thought he left and went on his way.

Later, after the shop was closed and the chores

done, John and Mary sat with their children around the table enjoying a good supper of hot chili. John related his conversation with Albert Martin.

"You know, if it is true that prayer and Bible reading are hindered by works of evil, I wonder more and more if this is our problem. But Albert also stated that prayer and Bible reading hinder the works of evil. This is certainly scriptural, for Jesus is the Christ, the Son of God who became victorious over sin, Satan, death, and hell. Therefore He has more power than Satan. Even though the Bible teaches that Satan is mighty, God is almighty."

"Do you think then," questioned Mary, "that prayer could answer if *braucha* really comes from God or not?"

"Yes, I definitely do," replied John, "and I think maybe we can find our answer soon. Do you remember last night when we were up with the twins how Aaron was biting his teeth together? That's a sign of parasites."

"Yes, I remember," Mary said thoughtfully. "His appetite isn't very good either. What do you have in mind?"

"Well," hesitated John, trying to fit his plan

together in his mind before he exposed it, "Old Jake goes by here every evening to Sam Beiler's to treat their baby, and I thought maybe I could have him stop in on his way home. Meanwhile, we should prepare with prayerful hearts, asking God to show us His will by praying that if this power isn't from Him, He won't let anything happen."

Chapter Four

Trying the Spirits

"There he comes now!" Mary pointed as she saw Jake through the window. John hurried out the front door and waved. Old Jake jerked his horse so suddenly that its feet slid on the pavement. After a while John came back in and said Jake would stop on his way back if it wasn't too late.

The rest of the evening was spent quietly and prayerfully. John found a place where he could be alone and prayed earnestly that God's will would be revealed. Mary rocked one of the twins, softly singing "Sweet Hour of Prayer."

Their thoughts were abruptly interrupted by a loud knock on the door. It opened, and Old Jake came hobbling in.

"Good evening," said John as he walked toward the kitchen to meet Jake. Jake seemed nervous and hurried as he walked on into the living room. "Which one is it tonight?" asked Jake.

"It's three-year-old Aaron," answered John, pointing to the small lad sitting on the rocking chair playing with a toy. "We think he may have some parasites, and we know you have treated children for that before."

Kneeling in front of the chair, Old Jake went through his usual motions, yet he appeared puzzled. After what seemed to John and Mary a long time, although it was probably only four or five minutes, Old Jake slowly stood up, shaking his bead in disbelief.

"I know he has parasites," he stated, "but I can't do anything for him. I don't understand. I have treated many children with parasites with good results, but . . ."

He left his sentence unfinished and slowly walked toward the door. John and Mary stood there looking at each other, reading each other's thoughts.

"Thanks for coming anyway," said John as Jake closed the door, still shaking his head.

Everything was quiet for a while, as John and Mary were lost in their own thoughts. Breaking the silence, John said, "I, ah, believe our prayers were answered, don't you?"

"Yes," answered Mary, still finding it hard to believe that God had answered so soon.

A week or so later John strode into the kitchen carrying a sack of groceries in each arm. After setting them on the table, he called Mary, saying, "Guess what Sam Beiler told me today in town." Not waiting for an answer, he went on. "You know Jake was going over every evening or so to give their baby a treatment. I guess he finally got tired of going over so often and told them he can just as well *brauch* for their baby at home without even seeing it. Sam said it seems to help just as much now as it did before, although he was a little skeptical and thought this might be going too far. He said Ben King on the other side of Greentown can *brauch*, but he does it differently than Old Jake.

Sam felt that maybe this is the more scriptural way of laying on hands."

Mary listened intently. "Do you think we should try it sometime?" she asked.

"Maybe we could go over tonight after supper," John replied. "We can do the same as we did when Jake was here the last time. Maybe Ben can help the twins' colic, if it really is laying on of hands."

John reached into his coat pocket. "Oh, by the way," he said, "I happened to find the book Albert was talking about the other day—*Between Christ and Satan*—in the bookstore today as I was browsing around. Maybe it can furnish us with some answers that the Bible isn't clear on." Laying the book on the table with the groceries, John went out to put his horse away and do chores.

A few hours later John and Mary were sitting in a small room just off the living room in Ben King's home. The family was still eating supper when John and Mary arrived, and Ben promised to be with them just as soon as they were done. This gave John and Mary the opportunity to pray.

"Do they both have colic?" inquired Ben as he entered the room, rubbing his hands as if they were cold. Closing the door after him, he took Ruth as Mary handed her to him.

"Yes," Mary answered, "although Ruth seems to have it worse than Ruby."

John and Mary sat silently, watching closely, their hearts pounding. Ben didn't make any peculiar motions as he cupped both hands around Ruth's stomach. Soon Ben and John were talking about the weather, the farm, the shop, and other material matters.

After a while Ben handed Ruth back to Mary. John gave Ruby to him, asking, "What would you call *braucha?*"

Looking up at John's question, Ben answered unhesitatingly, "Why, it is laying on of hands. You know the Bible talks about the gift of healing through laying on of hands."

"How did you discover that you had this gift?" questioned John.

"To make a long story short," said Ben, "I was cleaning the dirt off the alternator gauge glass on the power unit one day and noticed that the needle moved back and forth with my finger. We all have some magnetic force within us, only some are much stronger than others. I can even feel if someone near me in church has a headache. My head starts to hurt, and the other man's headache disappears.

"Well, here you go," said Ben, handing Ruby back to John. "It really doesn't seem to be real bad on either one." Reaching into his pocket, he pulled out a pack of cigarettes and lit one.

"Well, we must be going," remarked John. "What do we owe you?"

"There's a box over there. You can put in whatever you feel like," answered Ben.

Again as they were going down the road toward home, John and Mary were lost in their own thoughts. Finally Mary said, "I didn't know Ben smoked."

"I thought I could smell it when we walked into the house, but I didn't realize he was so open with it," replied John. "I don't understand how someone could have a gift of God, such as the gift of healing, yet live after the lusts of the flesh, such as smoking."

"It seems to me," mused Mary, "that to possess such a gift from God, one would need to be a born again believer, filled with the Holy Spirit."

John nodded. "Paul wrote in his epistle to Titus, 'the grace of God that bringeth salvation hath appeared to all men, teaching us that, denying ungodliness and worldly lusts, we should live soberly, righteously, and godly, in this present world.' This verse is not a very fitting description of most of the *braucha* I know of."

"What really is laying on of the hands then?" inquired Mary.

"I was just reading on that last night and found that this was usually done so that newly ordained apostles and ministers would receive the power of the Holy Spirit. We still do this when ordaining bishops. In none of the instances was it only for healing, although in Corinthians we read that there is a gift of healing. But it also talks about the gifts of prophecy, miracles, diverse tongues, and interpretation of tongues. Why do so many of our people claim to have the gift of healing, yet deny that any of the other gifts are available in our day and age?"

The next evening John was deeply engrossed in the book he had bought. "Mary!" he exclaimed suddenly. "Listen to this! A third elementary form of magic is based on magnetism or mesmerism. A man named Frank Mesmer discovered that he had a magnetic force in him with which he could heal people. He felt he could probably hypnotize. Scientifically they can't prove that it works, but then, science does not recognize supernatural forces as a source of power."

"Does the author say anything about how someone becomes involved in this magnetism?" asked Mary.

"Yes, he does," replied John. "He says most people who practice this inherit their power from ancestors who practiced it. This would stand to reason, for we all inherit a sin nature when we are born, and often our elders' greatest weakness becomes our hardest battle to overcome. For example, a man who has a quick temper is quite likely to have children with the same problem. It is very likely that I inherited this *braucha* power from my grandfather."

"Surely God wouldn't hold us responsible for the sins of our forefathers?" questioned Mary.

"No," John replied. "We are only accountable for our own sins. But we may have stronger tendencies toward certain sins that were practiced in former generations. And some learned behaviors might just be passed down."

"Lately you aren't able to quiet down the babies as well as you use to," observed Mary. "Do you think you have lost your power?"

"It seems so," answered John. "It was my prayer that, if this is an inherited evil, God would cleanse me through the blood of Jesus Christ and cleanse my heart from all desires for this power. I believe my prayer was answered."

In Search of Truth

Chapter Five

More Treatments

A few months later John visited his sister's place, where he helped with the butchering.

"I saw another kind of healing today," he told Mary when he got home. "This may be different than *braucha*. Maybe it's more like foot treatments. They claim you're treating the nerve endings, which are connected to the spot of your body ailment. They call this 'contact healing,' where they just hold their finger on a certain part of the body where supposedly there is a nerve ending."

"I don't know," Mary said skeptically. "But the twins are almost nine months old already, and we still get up three and four times a night with each of them. We've tried different formulas, medicine, goat's milk, and *braucha*. I guess I'm getting a little desperate!"

"Why don't we drive over there tonight," suggested John, "before we form an opinion."

A few hours later found them ushered into the living room with both babies, only to find they had to wait until Katie was done with another patient. After the other patient was gone, Katie motioned Mary and Ruth into another small room, where she twirled some kind of a stick between her hands. On top of the stick was an ugly, long-haired head. As she twirled this stick, the long hair stood straight out and sent shivers down Mary's back.

Katie spent a few minutes searching for the right spot on Ruth's abdomen. When she found it, she pressed her forefinger against the spot. Suddenly Katie started shaking her head violently every half minute or so, making terrible faces, as if something really hurt her. Mary sat there terrified, not knowing what to think. This was completely different from anything they had ever experienced.

After witnessing the same process with Ruby, John began asking questions.

"Can you tell us what's wrong with the twins?" inquired John.

"They both have stomachaches, probably colic," Katie concluded. "I would suggest you have them treated again day after tomorrow."

"How do you know where the certain spots are to hold your fingers?" inquired John.

"I just try different areas until I find the sore spot and then hold it until it goes away," Katie replied. "Some call this acupuncture without needles. It treats the nerve endings. I believe it is a gift from God."

"Why do you shake your head so vigorously?" asked John.

"That helps to work it off so I don't get sick as the pain is drawn out of the patient," answered Katie.

"Well," stalled John a little, not knowing if he should ask any more questions, "what about that little stick you twirl between your hands? What does that do?"

"That's really nothing," Katie replied. "It just helps replenish the drawing power. Anyone who *brauchs* needs to restore his power somehow."

"Thanks for your time," John replied as he got up to leave. "We'll see how the girls are until day after tomorrow. That will be Thursday."

Thursday evening came, and John wasn't sure what to do. He and Mary had discussed Katie's actions and had formed the opinion that it was probably another form of *braucha*. Yet they felt they should be sure, for Katie had assured them that it was a gift of God.

"Suppose I go alone and take Ruth with me," suggested John. "Katie thought she was worse than Ruby, though neither one is any better than she was. Lets pray fervently that God's will may be revealed to us."

This time John didn't need to wait. Katie took Ruth right away and went into her little room, leaving John alone in the living room. A curtain across the doorway prevented John from seeing what was going on.

Katie was soon back. "Are you sure this one was the worst?" she asked.

"Yes, I am sure," replied John.

"Well," sighed Katie, "I don't know what's wrong, but I can't find any sore places on her whole body. Are you sure she wasn't any better?"

"Yes, I am sure. We were up at least three times with her last night," answered John, relief flooding his soul as he realized that God had again answered his prayers.

After coming home and relating everything to Mary, they both felt compelled to kneel and thank their Maker for showing His will and for answering their prayers. Yet they still felt the emptiness of lacking a truly biblical way of healing.

A few months later something happened that filled that emptiness with God's wisdom.

Chapter Six

Real Answers

"Did you know Melvin Beiler had an accident?" John asked as he burst in the door. "I talked to Sovilla in the doctor's office today while I was waiting on a prescription." Melvin and his wife Sovilla were good friends of John and Mary's.

"What happened?" asked Mary as she stood by the table folding diapers.

"The horses ran away with the hay rake," John said. "Melvin was thrown under the rake and was bruised quite badly, although no bones were broken."

"Oh, my!" exclaimed Mary sympathetically. "He is a bleeder, isn't he?"

"Yes, he is," answered John. "That is what makes his condition so serious. Sovilla said the doctor told them that he has done everything he can for them. She just broke down and cried as she talked, and I felt so sorry for them."

"Is he at home?" Mary wondered.

"Yes. I thought we should go over one evening to visit them," John replied.

A week went by before John and Mary were able to get away. They had heard no more about Melvin's condition. Not knowing what to expect, they prepared themselves for the worst. Walking into the bedroom where Melvin was lying in bed with his feet elevated slightly, they were surprised how well he looked.

"How is it going?" John asked, shaking hands with Melvin.

"Quite well," Melvin answered, smiling.

"You must have made quite a change for the better," remarked John. "Last week I talked with Sovilla in the doctor's office and things didn't sound so good."

"Yes, after the doctor gave up on me, we decided God was the only one we could turn to. We asked the ministers to come that evening, as I felt I wanted to be anointed."

"I have often wondered about anointing with oil. I know James 5 speaks about it, yet it seems that mostly old people ask for it just before they expect to die. How is it done, anyway?" asked John.

"First the bishop asked me to examine my life very closely and confess any hidden or open sins, which I did. Then he said if there was anyone in the room who didn't believe with his whole heart that this was the scriptural method for healing, he should leave the room. Then everyone stood as the bishop led in prayer. After prayer he put some olive oil on his hand and anointed my head in the name of Jesus Christ for the healing of the body and soul according to His will."

"Do you believe that was what put you on the road to recovery?" asked John.

"There is no doubt in my mind," answered Melvin. "Although if it would not have been God's will to return my health, I would still feel the peace of mind I have since the anointing. It was the right thing to do."

"Would it be scriptural to anoint a child?" wondered John. He had never heard of anyone doing it.

"I don't believe it would be any more scriptural to anoint a child than it would be to baptize one," replied Melvin. "After all, a child has no sins to confess, nor can it have faith for healing."

Though it was late when they got home, John and Mary decided to study James 5 before they went to bed. As John found the verses he was looking for, he began reading out loud. " 'Is any sick among you? Let him call for the elders of the church; and let them pray over him, anointing him with oil in the name of the Lord.' What Melvin said tonight about his experience with anointing sure sounds scriptural so far, don't you think?" said John, looking up at Mary.

Mary nodded in agreement as John continued reading. " 'And the prayer of faith shall save the sick, and the Lord shall raise him up; and if he have committed sins, they shall be forgiven him.' Remember what Melvin said about the bishop asking anyone to leave the room if they didn't have faith?" John asked, getting more excited as he read on. " 'Confess your faults one to another, and pray for one another, that ye may be healed.'

"Here it talks about confessing our faults, just as Melvin explained it," John said thoughtfully. "Maybe this is one of the problems in our churches. It seems easier to find another's fault instead of confessing our own. Although I do believe we need discipline for church purity and for the good of our souls."

"I still wonder," pondered Mary after being silent all the while, "if anointing is for adult believers only. Is there nothing to do for children other than taking them to the medical doctor?"

"No, the doctor isn't the only thing left," pondered John. "Even though we should be thankful to God for the knowledge he has given to mankind for the benefit of man's health, it is still in God's hands to do His will and not ours. But lets finish verse 16, for I think this holds the real answer, if we would only use it more often. 'The effectual fervent prayer of a righteous man availeth much.' "

"You know," remarked Mary, a faraway look in her eyes, "if *braucha* really hinders prayer and Bible reading, is it any wonder that our churches are becoming so indifferent toward spiritual matters and so formal in prayer? Could this be another way Satan deceives us, by thinking it has been this way for a long time so we accept it as right regardless of whether or not we have scriptural support?"

"Yes, that could very well be true," John replied. "Although we need to be careful that we do not put too much emphasis on one point and forget something else the Bible teaches that's just as important. Our lives must always stay in balance with the Scriptures, and even then we confess that we fail in being consistent. May our confidence and trust always be in God's truth and not in our own understanding."